Answers and teaching explanations are on the
back of each question page

PASTEST REVISION BOOKS FOR MRCP 1

PasTest publish a wide range of revision books including:

MCQs in Basic Medical Sciences for MRCP 1
300 exam-based MCQs with answers and detailed explanatory notes

MRCP 1 Practice Exams: 2nd edition
Five complete MCQ Papers (300 MCQs) covering favourite Royal College topics

MRCP 1 MCQ Revision Book: 3rd edition
300 MCQs arranged by subject with correct answers and teaching notes, plus one complete mock exam

MRCP 1 Past Topics: A Revision Syllabus: 2nd edition
Contains authoritative lists of past topics which have occurred in the Royal College examination over the past 5 years

Explanations to the RCP Past Papers
Correct answers and teaching notes related to the Royal College Green and Blue books of actual past exam questions

MRCP Part 1 MCQs with Key Topic Summaries: 2nd edition
200 MCQs related to current examination syllabus with 200 comprehensive topic summaries

Membership at your Fingertips: MCQs on Disk
The disk contains 650 MCQs. Clear and concise teaching notes with every question

Oxford Textbook of Medicine MCQs: 3rd edition
375 new MCQs related to the 1995 Oxford Textbook of Medicine and ideal for subject based revision

For full details of all our revision books contact PasTest today on **01565 755226** for a free copy of our current book catalogue and price list. Books sent by return of post worldwide.

For full details contact:
**PasTest, Egerton Court, Parkgate Estate,
Knutsford, Cheshire WA16 8DX
Telephone 01565 755226 Fax 01565 650264**

INTRODUCTION

PasTest's MRCP Part 1 Pocket Books are designed to help the busy examination candidate to make the most of every opportunity to revise. With this little book in your pocket, it is the work of a moment to open it, choose a question, decide upon your answers and then check the answer on the back of the page. Revising "on the run" in this manner is both reassuring (if your answer is correct) and stimulating (if you find any gaps in your knowledge).

Each book contains 100 exam-based MCQs arranged by subject. Each author is a subject specialist who has based his selection of questions on past Royal College papers, and questions have also been designed specifically to address the basic sciences topics which have increasing prominence in the examination.

Each question consists of an initial statement followed by five possible completions, ABCDE. There is no restriction on the number of true or false items in a question. It is possible for all items in a question to be true or for all to be false. The four most important points of technique are:

1. Read the question carefully and be sure you understand it.
2. Mark your response clearly, correctly and accurately.
3. Use reasoning to work out your answer, but if you do not know the answer and cannot work it out, indicate "don't know".
4. The best possible way to obtain a good mark is to have as wide a knowledge as possible of the topics being tested in the examination.

It is possible to improve your mark by educated guessing, but this must be done with great care as incorrect answers are given a mark of −1 in the exam. You can use the books in this series to work out whether or not you are a good guesser by making a special mark against the responses that you have guessed before you check whether your responses are correct.

To get the best value from this book you should commit yourself to an answer for each item before you check the correct answer. With the answers on the back of each page, it can be tempting to find out which answers are correct before you have really decided on your own answer. But it is only by being sure of your own responses that you can ascertain which questions you would find difficult in the examination. Use the check boxes to mark your answers, or mark the parts of a question that you found difficult so that next time you look at the question you will be able to home in on your own personal areas of difficulty.

Books like the ones in this series, which consist of MCQs in subject categories, can help you to home in on specific topics and to isolate your weaknesses. You should plan a revision timetable to help you spread your time fairly over the range of subjects likely to appear in the examination. PasTest's *MRCP Part 1 Past Topics: A Revision Syllabus* will help you to work out which subjects deserve most of your revision time.

An effective revision plan should also include opportunities to practice your exam technique. Books of MCQ Practice Exams are indispensable and you should make time to sit at least two or three complete practice papers under timed conditions before the day of the actual examination arrives.

PasTest Revision Courses for MRCP 1

For 25 years PasTest, the leading independent specialists in post-graduate medical education, have been delivering top quality courses which have helped many thousands of doctors to pass the demanding MRCP Part 1 examination.

Our six-day MRCP Part 1 revision courses run three times each year at a convenient central London venue. Each delegate receives detailed course notes consisting of approximately 250 pages of exam-based MCQs with answers and comprehensive notes, plus many explanatory handouts.

> ✓ Learn from experienced and talented tutors with up-to-date knowledge of the requirements of the exam

> ✓ Teaching sessions focus on "favourite" exam topics and highlight possible areas of difficulty

> ✓ Four full practice exams enable you to constantly monitor your performance as the course progresses

For full details of the range of PasTest books and courses available for MRCP Part 1 candidates, contact PasTest today:

**PasTest, Egerton Court, Parkgate Estate,
Knutsford, Cheshire WA16 8DX
Telephone: 01565 755226 Fax: 01565 650264**

NEUROLOGY

Mark your answers with a tick (True) or a cross (False) in the box provided. Leave the box blank for 'Don't know'.

1. In Creutzfeldt Jacob disease (CJD)

- ☐ A 12% of cases are familial
- ☐ B increased CSF protein is often found
- ☐ C periodic sharp waves on the EEG are characteristic
- ☐ D cortical blindness may occur
- ☐ E death usually occurs within 12 months of onset

2. In Horner's syndrome

- ☐ A the pupil on the affected side will dilate with hydroxyamphetamine drops if the lesion is distal to the cervical ganglion
- ☐ B lateral medullary infarction is a recognised cause
- ☐ C the affected pupil dilates more widely than the normal one with phenylephrine drops if the lesion is preganglionic
- ☐ D the affected pupil fails to dilate with cocaine drops
- ☐ E injury to the upper trunks of the brachial plexus is a recognised cause

3. In multiple sclerosis

- ☐ A oligoclonal bands in the CSF and serum would not support the diagnosis
- ☐ B low amplitude visual evoked potentials would strongly support a demyelinating optic nerve lesion
- ☐ C prognosis is worse for men
- ☐ D onset with sensory symptoms heralds a good prognosis
- ☐ E beta-interferon decreases the relapse rate

Answers overleaf

1. **A C D E**

    CJD is a spongiform encephalopathy which usually presents as presenile dementia. 10–15% of cases are familial and onset is usually after the age of 50. Unsteadiness, memory and visual disturbance often occur early with progressive dementia, ataxia and upper motor neurone signs following. Myoclonus and aphasia may occur. CSF is usually normal and the EEG often shows periodic triphasic sharp waves. There is atrophy of most of the cortex with frontal, parietal and occipital lobes and cerebellum being worst affected. Recently a subgroup of CJD has been reported in much younger patients where psychiatric symptoms predominate early, leading to motor problems. There seem to be no characteristic EEG changes.

2. **B D**

    Horner's syndrome consists of mild ptosis, miosis and variable loss of sweating over the affected side of the face. The lesion may be central, preganglionic or postganglionic according to its site with respect to the superior cervical ganglion. Hydroxyamphetamine drops release noradrenaline from the terminal axon if this is functioning and therefore dilate the pupil of central or preganglionic Horner's but not of postganglionic Horner's (because the axon is no longer functioning). Phenylephrine dilates the normal and abnormal pupil equally in both central and preganglionic peripheral types of Horner's. However in postganglionic Horner's denervation hypersensitivity causes the affected pupil to dilate more widely than the normal side. Cocaine blocks the re-uptake of noradrenaline from the neuromuscular junction of the dilator muscle of the pupil, dilating the normal pupil. In any type of Horner's cocaine drops will not dilate the pupil of the affected eye, because noradrenaline is not being liberated into the nerve-muscle junction. The outflow of sympathetic innervation to the pupils is at T1 level and therefore Horner's syndrome may follow damage to the lower trunks of the brachial plexus.

3. **A C D E**

    Oligoclonal bands in the serum would suggest immunoglobulin production outside the CSF. Typically, visual evoked potentials are delayed (due to demyelination). Axonal loss would cause a decrease in amplitude. Prognosis is better in women and if the disease starts with optic or sensory symptoms. Increased age, progressive disease, spinal cord or cerebellar disease carry a poorer prognosis. Interferon has been shown to decrease the number and severity of relapses. Although some neurologists are sceptical of the trials these are the reasons why the drug has been given a licence in the UK.

4. Normal pressure hydrocephalus (NPH)

☐ A commonly presents with papilloedema with no focal signs

☐ B is characterised by the early onset of urinary incontinence

☐ C characteristically presents with dementia and gait disturbance

☐ D is demonstrable on CT scan by hydrocephalus with a normal sized fourth ventricle

☐ E may be improved by ventricular shunting

5. The following are true with regard to pyramidal weakness:

☐ A hip flexors are often weaker than knee flexors

☐ B ankle clonus is only present when the ankle jerks are brisk

☐ C wrist flexors will usually overcome wrist extensors

☐ D it may occur in the absence of any sensory signs

☐ E it is often present in syringomyelia

6. In motor neurone disease (MND)

☐ A sensory symptoms at onset do not exclude the diagnosis

☐ B peripheral sensory conduction velocities are normal

☐ C the function of the glossopharyngeal nerve is frequently affected

☐ D the onset of bulbar palsy indicates a poor prognosis

☐ E the abdominal reflexes are usually preserved

Answers overleaf

4. B C E

The classic clinical triad of NPH is dementia with early urinary incontinence and gait disturbance. Patients with NPH may not have these features but the CT scan appearance is often helpful since hydrocephalus is present with an enlarged fourth ventricle but normal or compressed cortical sulci (i.e. the pattern of communicating hydrocephalus). Many patients improve with ventricular shunting though prior CSF flow studies may be necessary to identify patients most likely to improve. If hydrocephalus is present with a normal sized fourth ventricle then the diagnosis is likely to be aqueduct stenosis or other obstructive lesion between the fourth and third ventricle. Papilloedema is not a feature of NPH.

5. A B C D E

In pyramidal weakness the flexors are usually stronger than the extensors in the upper limbs and the reverse in the lower limbs. Hip flexion is often weaker than ankle dorsiflexion which in turn is weaker than knee flexion. Ankle clonus and ankle jerks use the same L5 / S1 reflex pathway. Motor neurone disease, hereditary spastic paraparesis and parasagital meningiomas may all cause pyramidal weakness without sensory signs.

6. A B D E

Some patients have vague sensory symptoms in the early stages of MND and limb pain is a surprisingly frequent problem later in the disease. However sensory signs are never present. Essential to the diagnosis is the demonstration that the peripheral sensory conduction velocities are normal. The glossopharyngeal nerve is purely sensory and so is not affected in MND, thus severe bulbar problems may be present, but palatal sensation is normal. The prognosis for life in MND once bulbar symptoms develop is usually measured in months. The abdominal reflexes, which usually disappear in the face of upper motor neurone lesions, are often strangely preserved in MND, the explanation is unknown.

7. **With regard to the normal autonomic nervous system**
   - ☐ A 2.5% methacholine causes pupillary constriction
   - ☐ B the parasympathetic outflow to the ciliary muscle is via the superior colliculus
   - ☐ C beat to beat variations of the heart rate may be used to assess vagal integrity
   - ☐ D parasympathetic innervation of the bladder and lower bowel is via the dorsal nucleus of the vagus
   - ☐ E postganglionic sympathetic activity is mediated by noradrenaline

8. **Neurofibromatosis**
   - ☐ A may be complicated by carotid artery occlusion
   - ☐ B is associated with an increased incidence of cerebral microgliomas
   - ☐ C is suggested by the presence of more than five café-au-lait spots
   - ☐ D may be complicated by bilateral sensorineural deafness
   - ☐ E is inherited as an autosomal dominant characteristic

9. **In the spinal cord**
   - ☐ A inputs from the lumbar spine nerve roots lie medial to those from the thoracic region in the spinothalamic tracts
   - ☐ B a lesion of the anterior spinal artery will cause loss of pain sensation and hyperreflexia
   - ☐ C multiple sclerosis causes demyelination of the central grey matter
   - ☐ D syringomyelia may cause the same symptoms and signs as an ependymoma
   - ☐ E the posterior spinal artery is rarely damaged

Answers overleaf

7. **C E**

    2.5% methacholine causes pupillary constriction in denervated pupils (e.g. Holmes Adie). The superior colliculus is involved in gaze, the Edinger Westphal nucleus supplies the ciliary muscle. Heart rate changes in response to the Valsalva manoeuvre, deep breathing and posture are also used to assess autonomic innervation of the heart. The bladder, along with the genitalia and rectum, is innervated via the S2–4 parasympathetic nerves (S2,3,4 keep the wee off the floor!!). Preganglionic sympathetic and pre and post ganglionic parasympathetic nerves use acetylcholine as their neurotransmitter.

8. **A C D E**

    Neurofibromatosis is the commonest autosomal dominantly inherited neurocutaneous disorder. The hallmark of the disease is a combination of multiple pigmented 'café-au-lait' spots, cutaneous neurofibromas and plexiform neuromas. There is a tendency to develop schwannomas and neurofibromas on peripheral and cranial nerves. There may be bilateral acoustic neuromas and a tendency to develop cerebral astrocytomas, particularly optic gliomas. In children cerebrovascular occlusive disease including carotid occlusion may occur and hydrocephalus due to aqueduct stenosis is frequent. More than five 'café-au-lait' spots measuring 1.5 cm or more are suggestive of the diagnosis and axillary freckling is a characteristic feature. Further complications include phaeochromocytoma, Wilms' tumour and non-lymphocytic leukaemia.

9. **B D E**

    The somatotopic arrangement in the spinothalamic tract has the lower spinal roots more lateral. The anterior spinal artery supplies the anterior two-thirds of the cord including the spinothalamic tracts. Syringomyelia, ependymomas and central astrocytomas will all cause a central cord syndrome.

10. In the Guillain-Barré syndrome

☐ A sensory symptoms in the digits are a frequent early feature

☐ B the CSF cell count is frequently elevated in the first few days of the illness

☐ C the peak flow rate is the clearest guide to the need for artificial ventilation

☐ D limb ataxia frequently occurs in severely affected patients

☐ E there may be an underlying lymphoma

11. The following are correctly matched:

☐ A pineal tumours and hypopituitarism

☐ B expressive dysphasia and frontal lobe lesions

☐ C poor two point discrimination and a parietal lobe lesion

☐ D upper quadrantic homonymous hemianopia and a parietal lobe lesion

☐ E apraxia and a dominant parietal lobe lesion

12. Gait ataxia

☐ A is a sign of a cerebellar hemisphere lesion

☐ B may be the presenting feature of benign intracranial hypertension

☐ C is a presenting sign of cerebellar ectopia

☐ D occurs as a feature of carbamazepine toxicity

☐ E occurs in cerebellar vermis lesions

Answers overleaf

10. A B D E

Post-infective polyradiculopathy or the Guillain-Barré syndrome usually presents with sensory symptoms in the limbs followed by an ascending sensorimotor deficit. Severely affected cases show quite marked ataxia which cannot be entirely explained by joint-position loss and may be related to defective functioning of muscle spindle afferents. In the initial few days of symptoms the CSF cell count may be raised but later the classical pattern of high protein with a normal cell count appears. Ventilation may be impaired in severe cases in which the bulbar musculature is denervated and it is essential to monitor this. The test to use is the vital capacity, not the peak flow which is mainly a measure of airway size rather than ventilation volume. Uncommonly the Guillain-Barré syndrome may be the presenting feature of an underlying lymphoma.

11. A B C

Pineal tumours may be of many different cell types, the minority (25%) originating from pineal cells. Clinical features are from local pressure effects on the midbrain, aqueduct blockage of CSF and spread of cells through the 3rd ventricle causing hypothalamic damage (diabetes insipidus, hyper/hypophagia, precocious puberty and hypopituitarism) or optic chiasmal damage. Localisation of brain function is a common topic for MCQ questions. Broca's area is frontal, Wernicke's (receptive dysphasia) is temporal. Cortical sensation is a parietal lobe function (postcentral gyrus). Apraxia and agnosia are usually non-dominant parietal lobe functions.

12. C D E

Lesions in one or other cerebellar hemisphere usually cause peripheral limb ataxia (e.g. 'finger to nose ataxia') rather than ataxia of gait which is a feature of central cerebellar (vermis) lesions. Gait ataxia is associated with normal pressure hydrocephalus not benign intracranial hypertension. Cerebellar ectopia may present with a combination of gait ataxia and nystagmus (often downbeating vertically). Gait ataxia and other cerebellar signs are features of alcohol and anticonvulsant (including carbamazepine) toxicity.

13. The following are correctly matched:

☐ A biceps brachialis and the musculocutaneous nerve

☐ B internal rotation of the shoulder and teres minor

☐ C brachioradialis and the median nerve

☐ D elbow supination and a lateral movement of the thumb

☐ E pinching of thumb and index finger and the anterior interosseous nerve

14. In the carpal tunnel syndrome

☐ A there is increased latency of the median sensory action potential

☐ B wasting of the whole of the thenar eminence occurs

☐ C Tinel's sign is usually negative

☐ D there is delay in the median distal motor latency

☐ E in a severe case there will be weakness of extensor pollicis brevis

15. The following are true of the axillary plexus:

☐ A the radial nerve comes from the posterior cord

☐ B the median nerve comes from the medial cord alone

☐ C the ulnar nerve comes from the medial cord alone

☐ D a lesion of the axillary nerve causes sensory loss over the trapezius muscle

☐ E coracobrachialis is innervated by the musculocutaneous nerve

Answers overleaf

13. A B D E

Peripheral innervation is another common MRCP topic. Brachio-radialis is supplied by the musculocutaneous nerve. Supination is the movement of moving the hand from palm down to palm up; supinator, C6, radial nerve. Pronation is the opposite; pronator teres / pronator quadratis, C6, median. The anterior interosseous nerve is a branch of the median nerve given off just below the elbow. A lesion will give rise to weakness of the long flexors of the thumb and index finger.

14. A D

Tinel's sign is positive when tapping the wrist causes paraesthesia in the digits supplied by the median nerve. It is a sign of the carpal tunnel syndrome. Only three of the muscles of the thenar eminence are supplied by the median nerve, the abductor pollicis brevis, opponens pollicis and the flexor pollicis brevis. Prolongation of the latency of the sensory action potential is electrophysiological evidence of median nerve compression at the wrist, with progressive reduction of its amplitude as denervation occurs. Similarly the distal motor latency to median supplied muscles (abductor pollicis brevis is usually tested) is delayed in the face of normal motor conduction proximal to the wrist.

15. A C E

Posterior cord – Radial nerve (PR). Medial cord – Ulnar nerve (MU). Medial and Lateral cords – Median nerve (MLM). The axillary nerve (posterior cord C5–6) supplies deltoid and teres minor. A lesion causes weakness of shoulder abduction between 15 and 90 degrees and sensory loss over the anterior aspect of the shoulder. The musculocutaneous nerve (lateral cord C5–6) innervates biceps, brachialis and coracobrachialis (BBC) and skin over the outer border of the upper arm.

16. Huntington's chorea

- ☐ A is inherited as an autosomal recessive characteristic
- ☐ B may present with extrapyramidal rigidity in younger victims
- ☐ C always becomes clinically apparent by the third decade of life
- ☐ D is associated with loss of volume of the caudate nucleus on CT scans
- ☐ E usually responds to L-dopa therapy

17. The following are true:

- ☐ A C fibre activation usually causes a sharp pain
- ☐ B trigeminal neuralgia is best treated surgically
- ☐ C causalgia usually occurs after complete nerve transection
- ☐ D itch is C fibre mediated, unlike touch
- ☐ E sympathetic block with guanethidine is used in the treatment of some chronic pains

18. Vertical nystagmus

- ☐ A if upbeating, may indicate cerebellar tonsillar ectopia
- ☐ B may occur with phenytoin toxicity
- ☐ C if downbeating, indicates a lesion at the foramen magnum
- ☐ D when present in an unconscious patient indicates a thalamic lesion
- ☐ E may present with the symptom of oscillopsia

Answers overleaf

16. B D

Huntington's chorea is inherited as an autosomal dominant characteristic with near complete penetrance. However the age of onset varies and may be delayed until the fifth or sixth decade of life. In younger patients there may be marked extrapyramidal rigidity, such juvenile onset cases having usually inherited the Huntington's gene from their father rather than their mother. The volume of caudate nucleus can be reduced on CT scan but this is not a reliable test particularly early in the course of the disorder. L-dopa will worsen the choreic movements of patients with Huntington's, the therapy for which is tetrabenazine. Major tranquillisers in the phenothiazine and butyrophenone classes may be necessary in more severely hyperkinetic patients.

17. D E

A-delta fibres signal sharp pain. C fibres, the slowest conducting fibres, give rise to dull or burning pain; some carry the sensation of itch. Trigeminal neuralgia is usually treated successfully by carbamazepine. Causalgia usually occurs after partial nerve injury and along with other chronic pains may benefit from sympathetic blockade. This may be achieved by lesioning sympathetic ganglia (surgery or phenol) or by noradrenaline depletion of sympathetic nerve terminals by regional intravenous guanethidine.

18. B C E

Drug toxicity (for example with phenytoin) may cause nystagmus in all directions, horizontal and vertical. If the fast phase is downbeating the lesion is usually low in the medulla near the cervico-medullary junction. Masses at this site (or the congenital Arnold-Chiari malformation) may present with a combination of occipital pain, ataxia and downbeating nystagmus. There may or may not be an oscillopsia, a sensation of the visual field bouncing up and down, with the nystagmus. Nystagmus does not occur in unconscious patients since the fast phase appears to depend on intact hemisphere function. In an unconscious patient with a thalamic lesion the eyes may be deviated downwards.

19. The following inherited disorders are known to have triplet repeats as their genetic abnormality:

☐ A dystrophia myotonica

☐ B Huntington's chorea

☐ C fragile X syndrome

☐ D multiple system atrophy

☐ E Gerstmann's syndrome

20. Focal delta (slow) wave activity on EEG

☐ A is a common normal finding in adults

☐ B indicates the presence of a focal structural lesion

☐ C indicates the need for further investigation

☐ D is found after a major cerebral infarction

☐ E indicates the presence of epilepsy

21. The following are true with regard to speech:

☐ A complete aphonia may be due to a dominant parietal lobe lesion

☐ B spastic dysarthria is commonly due to middle cerebral artery occlusion

☐ C extrapyramidal disease may cause hyperkinetic speech

☐ D poliomyelitis will cause a pseudobulbar dysarthria

☐ E cerebellar 'ataxic' speech is usually due to a vermis lesion

Answers overleaf

19. A B C

Triplet repeats have been shown as the genetic abnormality in a number of diseases. The number of repeats increases with subsequent generations and is thought to be the mechanism underlying 'anticipation' where succeeding generations inherit a more severe form of the disease. Gerstmann's syndrome occurs in some patients with parietal lobe damage (confusion between right and left limbs, finger agnosia, acalculia and agraphia).

20. B C D

Focal delta wave activity, particularly if continuous, suggests the presence of a structural brain lesion, but is pathologically non-specific and may occur after substantial vascular lesions of any type, tumours or even advanced neurodegenerative disease. Neurophysiologically this abnormality represents an area of electrically inactive cortex which allows the appearance on the surface EEG of underlying slow waves probably originating from the thalamic rhythm generators. The appearance of focal delta wave activity is an indication for further investigation by CT scanning. Although seizures may occur with such structural lesions the EEG appearances are not synonymous with clinical seizures, focal slow waves being seen in many patients with comparable structural lesions who have not had seizures.

21. B C E

Aphonia refers to noise production which may still be present with a parietal lesion. Spastic dysarthria is caused by upper motor neurone lesions which are commonly due to stroke, tumour or motor neurone disease. Extrapyramidal disease (Parkinson's / Huntington's chorea) may cause fast speech although hypokinetic speech is more common. Polio causes a lower motor neurone therefore bulbar dysarthria.

22. A tremor of the outstretched hands

☐ A is characteristic of Parkinson's disease

☐ B responds to propranolol

☐ C is often familial and benign

☐ D may be worsened by anxiety

☐ E is improved by primidone

23. In muscular dystrophies

☐ A the Becker dystrophy is X linked

☐ B Duchenne dystrophy may be seen in Turner's syndrome

☐ C cardiac involvement is usually subclinical in Becker dystrophy

☐ D pseudohypertrophy occurs in 80% of Duchenne muscular dystrophy (DMD)

☐ E EMG is useful in detecting female carriers

24. After a major cerebral infarction

☐ A a CT scan usually shows a low attenuation area within 2 hours

☐ B the unenhanced scan may be normal in the second week

☐ C contrast enhancement on the CT scan is maximal in the second week

☐ D a mass effect from ischaemic oedema is seen on the CT scan in the first 6 hours

☐ E carotid arteriography may be normal

Answers overleaf

22. B C D E

The tremor of Parkinson's disease is characteristically a rest tremor, though a mild action tremor is sometimes seen. Action tremors are usually an exaggeration of the normal physiological tremor, and like many tremors are worsened by anxiety. A marked action tremor may run in families and is seldom suggestive of serious neurological disease. Titubation of the head which is common in the elderly, is an action tremor of the neck muscles, is not a sign of Parkinson's disease and is usually benign but sometimes related to lesions of the superior cerebellar peduncle. The drug of first choice for troublesome action tremors is propranolol but in patients in whom this drug is ineffective or contraindicated, low doses of primidone may be effective.

23. A B D

DMD and Becker dystrophy are X-linked recessive, therefore males suffer the disease and females carry it unless the good X chromosome is missing (Turner's 45XO) or turned off (lyonisation) when the phenotype will be expressed. Becker dystrophy usually starts later, is less common and progresses slower than the other dystrophies. Cardiac muscle is spared and therefore there is not even subclinical involvement! Pseudo-hypertrophy results from fatty infiltration, the gastrocnemius, quadriceps, deltoid and tongue being most affected. Mean IQ is 10–20 points lower in Duchenne but normal in Becker; Duchenne and Becker are allelic variants. EMG is not helpful in detecting female carriers but creatine kinase estimation is.

24. B C E

Up to the first 12 hours or so after even a substantial cerebral infarction the CT scan may show very little change. In fact the extent of the low attenuation area caused by an infarction usually does not become clear for at least 12 hours and sometimes longer. Over the first 24–36 hours the ischaemic tissue swells, producing a mass effect on the scan by the second or third day which then subsides by the first week. Towards the end of the first week the infarcted tissue is invaded by phagocytic glial cells which may increase the X-ray attenuation of the area so that the plain scan looks (near) normal. However the infarct is also invaded by new blood vessels which show as areas of enhancement after injection of iodinated contrast medium. This post-contrast enhancement is maximal during the second week after the infarction. Carotid angiography after cerebral infarction may be normal even after substantial infarction. This occurs particularly following embolism when the causative occlusion may disperse. In such cases the longer after the stroke the angiogram is performed the more likely it is to be normal.

25. With inflammatory myopathies

☐ A muscles are tender in the majority of cases

☐ B dermatomyositis usually has a more acute onset than polymyositis

☐ C in dermatomyositis, excessive discoloration of the skin implies an underlying malignancy

☐ D cardiac muscle may be involved

☐ E extraocular muscles may be involved

26. After aneurysmal subarachnoid haemorrhage (SAH)

☐ A the syndrome of inappropriate ADH secretion may occur

☐ B the peak risk for secondary ischaemic complications is immediately after the haemorrhage

☐ C the risk of rebleeding is maximal in the month following the stroke

☐ D a catecholamine surge can cause direct myocardial damage

☐ E if the patient is comatose, referral for early aneurysm clipping is generally advised

27. CSF pleocytosis with normal CSF glucose is often seen in

☐ A TB meningitis

☐ B chronic meningeal fungal infection

☐ C multiple sclerosis

☐ D Guillain-Barré syndrome

☐ E torticollis

Answers overleaf

25. A B D

Polymyositis and dermatomyositis are very similar. Muscles are often painful although onset of weakness may be painless. Dermato-myositis is usually more acute and severe. It is associated with malignancy, the percentage with underlying malignancy being about the same as the patient's age (age 50, 50%, age 70, 70% etc.). Extraocular muscles are typically spared.

26. A C D

Hypothalamic damage frequently occurs after substantial SAH due to berry aneurysms. This causes excessive ADH secretion and is probably the cause of the surge of catecholamines which may cause life-threatening cardiac arrhythmias and subendocardial myocardial necrosis. There is usually a delay of some days (with a peak incidence in the second week) after SAH before secondary ischaemic changes become apparent. The risk of rebleeding, compared with deterioration due to vasospasm, has probably been overestimated and falls fairly sharply from up to 50% within the first month (in unoperated patients) such that at six months it is 3% per year. In general neurosurgeons do not consider aneurysmal clipping in patients who are unconscious since the outlook for such patients is so poor. Referral for such surgery is therefore delayed until the clinical condition of the patient has improved (provided that the diagnosis is clear).

27. C

Increased white cells and low glucose are seen in combination in TB meningitis, chronic infections and malignant meningitis. Be careful to read the question carefully to avoid making silly mistakes and losing marks!

28. Benign intracranial hypertension (BIH)

- ☐ A may present with transient visual obscurations
- ☐ B is a complication of anorexia nervosa
- ☐ C is associated with enlarged cerebral ventricles on CT scan
- ☐ D may complicate vitamin D toxicity
- ☐ E is treated by repeated lumbar puncture

29. The following are good prognostic indicators in head injury:

- ☐ A low Glasgow coma scale 24 hours after injury
- ☐ B presence of a skull fracture
- ☐ C history of alcohol consumption
- ☐ D absent somatosensory evoked responses
- ☐ E high cerebral blood flow 48 hours post injury

30. Extrapyramidal rigidity may be caused by

- ☐ A butyrophenone tranquillisers
- ☐ B B12 deficiency
- ☐ C abuse of synthetic pethidine derivatives
- ☐ D carbon monoxide poisoning
- ☐ E the neuroleptic malignant syndrome

Answers overleaf

28. A E

Despite raised pressure causing papilloedema BIH is a syndrome in which consciousness is clear and there are no focal neurological signs (although false localising signs such as sixth nerve palsies may occur). It may present with headache and transient visual obscurations which forewarn of visual failure. The cerebral ventricles are normal or smaller than usual, i.e. hydrocephalus is not present. BIH is not a feature of anorexia nervosa but occurs in young obese females often with menstrual irregularities. Other causes include pregnancy, the contraceptive pill, hypocortisolism, hypoparathyroidism, hyper- and hypovitaminosis A, tetracycline therapy and other drugs. Usually BIH is a self-limiting condition but because of the risk of visual loss, treatment with repeated lumbar puncture is advised. Steroids and carbonic anhydrase inhibitors have been suggested but are not usually effective.

29. A B D

Note the question asks for good prognostic indicators not indicators of a good prognosis! Low coma scale, skull fracture and absent somato-sensory evoked responses are all good indicators of a poor prognosis.

30. A C D E

Phenothiazine and butyrophenone tranquillisers block the D2 dopamine receptors in the corpus striatum and are the principal causes of iatrogenic Parkinsonism. In the early 1980s, a severe Parkinsonian syndrome appeared in Californian drug addicts caused principally by 1-methyl-4-phenyl-1,2,5,6-tetrahydropyridine (MPTP), a by-product of synthetic opiate manufacture. This has provided experimental oppor-tunities to understand the pathogenesis of idiopathic Parkinson's disease. In particular the possible role of monoamine oxidase B inhibitors in preventing the conversion of MPTP to MPP+ which is responsible for the substantia nigra neuronal damage raises the possibility of new treatments to prevent progress of the disease. The neuroleptic malignant syndrome is a rare, life-threatening complication of neuroleptic therapy which may also follow withdrawal from amantidine. Features include hyperpyrexia, severe extrapyramidal rigidity and autonomic disturbances. Treatment is by withdrawal of the neuroleptic drug and administration of dantrolene and/or bromocriptine.

31. Trigeminal neuralgia

- [ ] A if associated with multiple sclerosis (MS), often has no trigger spots
- [ ] B if associated with MS may be difficult to treat
- [ ] C may respond to phenytoin
- [ ] D is more common in patients with causalgia
- [ ] E if secondary to nerve compression is usually caused by root entry zone nerve damage

32. In a young person with an internuclear ophthalmoplegia

- [ ] A oligoclonal bands in the CSF confirm the diagnosis of multiple sclerosis
- [ ] B unilateral delay in the visual evoked potentials is strong evidence of the diagnosis of multiple sclerosis
- [ ] C the presence of extrinsic brain stem compression is indicated
- [ ] D high doses of intravenous steroids will speed recovery if demyelination is the cause
- [ ] E the lesion is in the median longitudinal fasciculus in the brain stem

33. The following are true with regard to neurosyphilis:

- [ ] A clinical neurological manifestations occur in about 10% of patients infected with *Treponema pallidum*
- [ ] B active disease is usually marked by oligoclonal bands in the CSF
- [ ] C a positive VDRL is specific
- [ ] D a large gumma will give symptoms of an intracranial tumour
- [ ] E 25% of neurosyphilis cases have tabes dorsalis

Answers overleaf

31. A B C E

Trigeminal neuralgia, whilst usually idiopathic may be secondary to demyelination (in the pons), in which case trigger spots are rare and treatment is often ineffective. Phenytoin, carbamazepine and clonazepam are the usual medical treatments. There is no association with causalgia except the pain mechanism may be similar. Root or root entry zone compression may occur due to tumours or arteries.

32. B D E

The diagnosis of multiple sclerosis depends on the demonstration of central nervous system lesions disseminated in time and place. An internuclear ophthalmoplegia is a sign of an intrinsic brain stem lesion affecting the median longitudinal fasciculus. If the spinal fluid is shown to contain gammaglobulin in an oligoclonal pattern it is very likely that multiple sclerosis is the cause. However oligoclonal bands are present in many other intrathecal inflammatory diseases and do not make multiple sclerosis certain. If delayed latency in the visual evoked response is demonstrated in a patient with an internuclear ophthalmoplegia, then more than one lesion is present and multiple sclerosis is probable. If there is a past history of optic neuritis the diagnosis is confirmed. In acute central nervous system demyelination due to multiple sclerosis, high dose intravenous steroids have been shown to shorten the duration of relapses though they probably have no effect on long-term disability.

33. A B D E

In neurosyphilis, the distinction between tertiary meningovascular (cerebrospinal) syphilis and tabes/general paresis is clinical. Meningovascular syphilis may affect any part of the nervous system by causing a pachymeningitis or endarteritis. CSF is usually abnormal with raised protein, immunoglobulin synthesis and oligoclonal bands. Tabes dorsalis by definition is atrophy of the dorsal spinal roots and posterior columns of the spinal cord including cranial nerve roots.

34. In a patient with diplopia

☐ A the paretic eye carries the most peripheral of the two images

☐ B retained capacity of the eye to intort indicates a superior oblique palsy

☐ C if the eye is deviated down and out the third cranial nerve is involved

☐ D failure of the eye to abduct indicates a fourth cranial nerve palsy

☐ E the lateral rectus is weak if the adducted eye cannot be depressed

35. Central pontine myelinolysis

☐ A is confined to the pons

☐ B is associated with Wernicke's encephalopathy

☐ C is associated with altered consciousness

☐ D is a cause of bulbar palsy

☐ E may relapse spontaneously

36. The following are features of tuberose sclerosis:

☐ A café-au-lait patches of pigmentation

☐ B ocular telangiectasias

☐ C cardiac rhabdomyomas

☐ D cerebral gliomas

☐ E cerebral aqueduct stenosis

Answers overleaf

34. A C

When assessing the cause of diplopia the first task is to determine which eye is involved. The cover test is the simplest method. Each eye is covered in turn while the patient is looking in the direction which causes most marked diplopia. When the paretic eye is covered, the most peripheral of the two images will disappear. The diplopia will be maximal in the direction of gaze produced by the paretic muscle. The main action of the superior oblique muscle is to depress the adducted eye. Adduction is not possible with a third nerve palsy and the eye is usually deviated down and out by the effect of the still intact muscles lateral rectus (sixth cranial nerve) and superior oblique (fouth cranial nerve). In a third nerve palsy, the action of the intact superior oblique can be seen by its secondary action of intorsion of the eye (watch a conjunctival blood vessel whilst the patient tries to look at the tip of his nose).

35. B C D

Central pontine myelinolysis (CPM) occurs when there is demyelination of the pons or parapontine white matter. It is due to metabolic insults and is seen in alcoholics, leukaemia, hyperemesis gravidarum and other causes of prolonged vomiting. It is therefore associated with Wernicke's. A flaccid paralysis and eye movement disorders are common findings. Recovery depends on the treatment of the underlying disease and relapse of CPM does not occur unless there is relapse of the underlying cause.

36. A C D

The classical lesions of tuberose sclerosis are adenoma sebaceum, red-brown papules in the butterfly distribution on the face, 'ash leaf' hypopigmented patches, and 'shagreen patches', usually over the lumbosacral area. However about 10% of patients have café-au-lait patches of pigmentation. Other CNS manifestations include epilepsy in association with cerebral malformations known as tubers and mental retardation. About 5% of children with tuberose sclerosis develop cerebral gliomas. Renal malformations may occur and cardiac rhabdomyomas are present in up to one-third of patients.

37. Regarding paraneoplastic syndromes

- ☐ A progressive cerebellar degeneration is associated with vitamin E deficiency
- ☐ B anti-Purkinje cell antibodies are associated with ovarian carcinoma
- ☐ C retinal degeneration is more common than optic nerve degeneration
- ☐ D pituitary release of ADH may cause the syndrome of inappropriate ADH secretion
- ☐ E Cushing's syndrome secondary to ectopic ACTH does not cause myopathy

38. In a right-sided hypoglossal nerve palsy

- ☐ A the protruded tongue will deviate towards the left
- ☐ B the soft palate will deviate towards the right
- ☐ C if the neighbouring three cranial nerves are involved, the lesion is likely to be in the region of the jugular foramen
- ☐ D taste will be impaired over the anterior two-thirds of the tongue
- ☐ E sensation will be impaired over the right side of the soft palate

39. In the lower limbs

- ☐ A the femoral nerve arises from L2,3,4 nerve roots
- ☐ B the sciatic nerve forms the tibial and common peroneal nerves
- ☐ C the tibial nerve supplies the gastrocnemius and soleus muscles
- ☐ D a complete sciatic nerve lesion will cause sensory loss over the hamstrings
- ☐ E a common peroneal nerve lesion will cause weakness of eversion of the foot

Answers overleaf

37. B C

There are many paraneoplastic syndromes. Cerebellar degeneration is associated with anti-Purkinje cell antibodies (secondary to breast and ovary tumours). Vitamin E deficiency does cause a cerebellar degeneration but this is not paraneoplastic. Optic atrophy is secondary to retinal degeneration in this case. SIADH is due to an ADH like peptide release from the tumour and Cushing's syndrome, whatever the cause, may have a myopathy.

38. C

The twelfth cranial nerve or hypoglossal nerve innervates the musculature of the tongue. Paralysis of this musculature on one side causes the protruded tongue to be pushed over towards the weak side. The soft palate obtains its sensory innervation from the ninth (glossopharyngeal) cranial nerve and its motor innervation from the (tenth nerve) vagus. A combination of lesions on one side of cranial nerves 9, 10, 11 and 12 suggests that the lesion is at the jugular foramen just outside the skull, for example a glomus tumour. Taste over the anterior two-thirds of the tongue is supplied by fibres which run in the facial nerve.

39. A B C E

In the lower limb the sciatic nerve supplies motor to the hamstrings and short head of biceps as well as forming the tibial and common peroneal nerves. Sensory supply is purely below the knee. The tibial nerve supplies gastrocnemius, popliteus, plantaris and soleus, tibialis posterior, flexor digitorum longus and flexor hallucis longus before becoming the medial and lateral plantar nerves (small muscles of the foot). The common peroneal nerve: superficial branch – peroneus longus and brevis; deep branch – tibialis anterior, extensor digitorum longus and brevis, extensor hallucis longus and peroneus.

40. After intervertebral disc prolapse

☐ A sensory loss is accompanied by reduced sensory action potentials in the relevant root distribution

☐ B pain is felt in the muscles innervated by the damaged nerve root

☐ C in the lumbar region an extensor plantar response may occur

☐ D in the lumbar region loss of bladder function may result

☐ E loss of the ankle reflex indicates an S1 root lesion

41. In lacunar syndromes

☐ A diagnosis is based on clinical signs

☐ B about half are pure motor strokes

☐ C ataxic hemiparesis may occur

☐ D visual field defects occur in about 30%

☐ E visuospatial disturbance should not be present in order to make the diagnosis

42. Muscle fasciculations

☐ A occur with reinervation of partially denervated muscles

☐ B in the calf muscles are often benign

☐ C may be seen during an edrophonium test for myasthenia gravis

☐ D are diagnostic of motor neurone disease (MND)

☐ E occur in spinal muscular atrophy

Answers overleaf

40. B D E

The dorsal root ganglia of the spinal roots are in the exit foramina of the spine. Compression by an intervertebral disc usually occurs proximal to this site and therefore the sensory action potential in the distal neurone is intact. Nerve root compression often causes pain which is felt in the muscles supplied by that segment, for example in the pectoralis muscle and triceps in a C7 root compression. Compression in the lumbar region cannot cause upper motor signs since the spinal cord ends at L1. A large central disc in the lower lumbar region may compress the sacral roots in the cauda equina and cause bladder symptoms. The root innervation of the ankle reflex is S1 so compression of this root will cause loss of the ankle jerk.

41. A B C E

Lacunar syndromes are predictive of small deep lesions in the motor (50%) and sensory (5%) pathways (mixed 35%). Most are due to small infarcts seen best on MRI. Higher cortical function loss is not a feature of lacunar syndromes. Ataxic hemiparesis occurs in about 10% and is the combination of corticospinal and ipsilateral cerebellar signs.

42. A B C E

Fasciculations consist of spontaneous contractions of single motor units visible to the naked eye. They are frequently seen in the quadriceps and calf muscles of healthy individuals and by themselves are not diagnostic of MND. In the latter disease the fasciculations are seen in many more muscles and are associated with wasting, weakness and other features of MND. Fasciculations may occur pathologically in many situations where there is partial denervation (e.g. root lesions). The origin is probably in the electrical instability of the reinervation (and excessive sensitivity to acetylcholine) that occurs in chronic partial denervation. Though not frequently seen in spinal muscular atrophy, fasciculations may occasionally be found in adult onset cases.

43. In the treatment of headache

☐ A sumatriptan is an analgesic

☐ B sumatriptan should only be given within two hours of a migraine attack

☐ C methysergide may cause obstructive nephropathy

☐ D long-acting beta blockers are often helpful in migraine

☐ E ergot derivatives no longer have a role in migraine management

44. Myasthenia gravis

☐ A is caused by autoantibodies directed against acetylcholine

☐ B in older men responds to thymectomy, especially if a thymoma is present

☐ C responds to high dose steroid therapy

☐ D may be worsened by aminoglycoside antibiotics

☐ E may be treated by long-term edrophonium therapy

45. In AIDS

☐ A CNS lymphoma is common

☐ B herpes simplex and herpes zoster are common

☐ C cerebral atrophy occurs

☐ D peripheral neuropathy occurs in about 20%

☐ E myopathy may be induced by zidovudine

Answers overleaf

43. C D

Sumatriptan affects blood flow by decreasing cerebral vasodilatation. It may be given at any stage of a migraine but should be avoided in combination with ergot, which still has a small part to play in management. Methysergide may cause retroperitoneal fibrosis and patients should be free from it for at least 3 months a year.

44. C D

The pathogenic mechanism in myasthenia gravis is the production of autoantibodies directed against the acetylcholine receptors on the motor end plate. These are present in 90% of patients with myasthenia although their titre correlates poorly with the clinical severity of the disease. Myasthenia in younger women is usually not associated with thymoma and responds well to thymectomy (some have recommended this as the first line of therapy in patients fit for operation). Older men with myasthenia are most likely to have a thymoma: it is present in about 10% of patients. Thymectomy is advised for such patients with thymoma because of the risks of local tumour infiltration but it usually has a disappointing effect on the myasthenia. Aminoglycoside antibiotics can worsen neuromuscular transmission in patients with myasthenia and may provoke onset. Pharmacological therapy of myasthenia is with long-acting anticholinesterase inhibitors, neostigmine and pyridostigmine. Edrophonium is too short acting for therapeutic use and is reserved for diagnostic purposes only.

45. A B C D E

In AIDS primary neural damage may occur causing atrophy. Secondary infection or tumours are also common. Myopathy secondary to zidovudine is clinically indistinguishable from AIDS myopathy.

46. A macular sparing hemianopia

- ☐ A indicates a lesion in the optic radiation
- ☐ B indicates a vascular lesion in the parietal lobe
- ☐ C does not prevent a patient from reading
- ☐ D will exclude a patient from holding a driving license
- ☐ E suggests a lesion in the posterior cerebral artery territory

47. The following are true:

- ☐ A meningiomas enhance with contrast on CT scans
- ☐ B T1 weighted MR scans are useful in diagnosing multiple sclerosis
- ☐ C a T1 nerve root lesion is often diagnosed by plain X-ray examination
- ☐ D PET scanning can pick up blood flow changes over a few milliseconds
- ☐ E functional MRI is now the investigation of choice for carotid stenosis

48. In Bell's palsy

- ☐ A the majority recover without residual weakness
- ☐ B a complete facial weakness is a poor prognostic sign
- ☐ C if the palsy is complete, tarsorrhaphy is usually required to protect the cornea
- ☐ D mild sensory symptoms at onset are a common feature
- ☐ E electrophysiological tests may be helpful prognostically

Answers overleaf

46. C D E

The macular region of the visual cortex is at the tip of the occipital lobe on its medial aspect and is supplied with blood by both the middle and posterior cerebral arteries. The result is that an infarction in the posterior cerebral artery territory causes a homonymous hemianopia which spares the macular region. Patients can usually read with this deficit since the ability to scan is retained. Lesions which interrupt the optic radiation in the parietal lobe cause a hemianopia which involves the macula and there are often visuoperceptual deficits which interfere with the ability to read. A patient with a visual field defect below the horizon of vision is not permitted to hold a driving licence.

47. A B

In T1 weighted images the CSF is black. Demyelinating plaques are easily seen. A T1 nerve root lesion due to an apical lung tumour or a cervical rib may show on a plain X-ray. However, most T1 lesions have other causes. PET scans need changes in blood flow for several tens of seconds for accurate localisation. Angiography remains the 'gold standard' for investigating carotid stenosis.

48. A B D E

The unilateral lower motor neurone palsy of unknown origin known as Bell's palsy is often preceded by pain in the mastoid region. At least 80% of cases show complete recovery but total paralysis at onset is a poor prognostic sign. In the latter case recovery does occur but cross re-inervation may produce unsatisfactory results. Tarsorrhaphy to protect the cornea is hardly ever necessary in Bell's palsy, though a supply of artificial tears (hydroxymellose drops) may be necessary. Corneal sensation is always intact and the uprolling of the eye to blink (the Bell's phenomenon) is usually sufficient protection of the cornea before spontaneous recovery occurs. After about three weeks, if recovery has not occurred EMG tests may help predict prognosis. If there is no evidence of denervation the prognosis for recovery is good.

49. After a single unprovoked seizure in adult life

- ☐ A a patient should not drive for one year
- ☐ B a normal EEG excludes epilepsy
- ☐ C life-long anticonvulsants are usually started
- ☐ D an EEG within 24 hours will usually show signs of epilepsy
- ☐ E a cerebral tumour is the most likely cause

50. Infarction in the territory of the anterior cerebral artery

- ☐ A causes more severe hand than shoulder weakness on the affected side
- ☐ B produces predominant weakness of the lower limb
- ☐ C is most frequently seen after subarachnoid haemorrhage due to berry aneurysm rupture
- ☐ D causes transcortical motor aphasia when affecting the dominant hemisphere
- ☐ E usually occurs as a result of cerebral embolism

Answers overleaf

49. A D

A single seizure does not constitute epilepsy. However, there is a 40–80% chance of a further seizure within 12 months. An EEG within 24 hours of a fit will show non-specific slowing. A normal EEG does not exclude the diagnosis of epilepsy nor does a normal CT exclude the possibility of a structural (e.g. small CVA) cause. After a single unprovoked seizure driving is banned for one year. If more than one fit occurs driving is banned for one year after the last fit whether the patient is on or off treatment. If all seizures occur during sleep (during sleep not just at night!) and that pattern has been set for three years driving is allowed. The commonest cause of epilepsy in adult life is cerebrovascular disease.

50. B C D

Anterior cerebral artery territory infarction is very uncommon in primary occlusive cerebrovascular disease and is almost always caused by secondary vasospasm following subarachnoid haemorrhage. Infarction in this territory causes predominant weakness of the lower limb and the proximal upper limb (the shoulder). The hand may be weakened by damage to the underlying fibres of the internal capsule but is less severely affected. Language function may be involved if the dominant hemisphere is damaged and this aphasia is characterised by a non-fluent aphasia (reduced word output) with good understanding and preserved ability to repeat words (transcortical motor aphasia). Damage to the anterior cerebral artery territory due to cerebral embolism is almost unheard of.

PSYCHIATRY

Mark your answers with a tick (True) or a cross (False) in the box provided. Leave the box blank for 'Don't know'.

51. In schizophrenia

☐ A the age of onset is on average 5 years earlier in females

☐ B outcome is better in developed compared with non-developed countries

☐ C the risk of developing the disorder is higher amongst lower social class families

☐ D the 'expressed emotion' of close family members is predictive of relapse

☐ E functional deterioration usually continues insidiously over the whole illness course

52. Fragile X syndrome is associated with the following features:

☐ A autosomal dominant inheritance

☐ B male predominance

☐ C bat ears

☐ D the possibility of antenatal detection

☐ E hyperkinetic syndrome

53. Typical features of obsessive-compulsive neurosis include

☐ A ruminations

☐ B family history of neurosis

☐ C rituals

☐ D progression to schizophrenia

☐ E resistance

Answers overleaf

51. D

Onset of schizophrenia, usually between 15 and 45 years of age, occurs on average five years earlier in males (median onset 28 years). One third of patients have a good or fair outcome and 10–20% a severe chronic illness. Deterioration in function usually plateaus after 3–5 years and florid symptoms often reduce with increasing age. Outcome is worse in developed countries, although incidence and symptomatology is similar worldwide. Increased prevalence within socio-economically deprived areas is due to downward 'social drift' after illness onset. High 'expressed emotion' in family members, particularly those with more than 35 hours per week contact with the patient, is highly predictive of relapse.

52. B C D E

Fragile X syndrome has been recognised in recent years as the commonest cause of X-linked mental retardation. The cardinal features are male sex, facial abnormalities (bat ears, large jaw, maxillary hypoplasia) macro-orchidism and a marker (an apparent gap in the long arm of the X-chromosome) in lymphocytic culture under reducing conditions. This marker can be seen in amniotic fluid cells and therefore prenatal diagnosis is possible. Carrier females are usually of normal intelligence, but about 10% have mild mental retardation. Recent reports have suggested high rates of infantile autism and hyperkinetic syndrome.

53. A C E

The key feature of an obsessional symptom is that the patient feels compelled to think or act in a certain way (compulsion) he recognises as absurd and attempts to resist (resistance). Ruminations are repetitive internal arguments about simple actions. Rituals are repeated irrational patterns of behaviour. There is probably a hereditary component in the aetiology of the condition but this is probably very small. The superficial similarity of obsessional symptoms and some of the features of schizophrenia is deceptive: there is no association between these two conditions.

54. In systemic lupus erythematosus (SLE)

☐ A cerebral manifestations occur in less than 10% of cases

☐ B schizophreniform psychosis is the commonest psychiatric manifestation

☐ C psychiatric symptoms are almost always due to cerebral arteritis

☐ D psychiatric symptoms usually precede fever and arthralgia

☐ E cerebral involvement is an indicator of poor prognosis

55. The following statements about alcohol dependence are true:

☐ A withdrawal symptoms typically occur in the morning

☐ B the commonest withdrawal symptoms are perceptual disturbances

☐ C most alcohol-dependent patients develop liver cirrhosis

☐ D intensive counselling has a significant effect on outcome

☐ E chlormethiazole deters impulsive drinking via the acetaldehyde reaction

56. The following factors increase the risk of psychiatric sequelae to head injury:

☐ A prolonged retrograde amnesia

☐ B a family history of mental disorder

☐ C the complete absence of post-traumatic amnesia

☐ D younger age

☐ E where the circumstances of the injury prohibit compensation

Answers overleaf

54. E

CNS involvement occurs in about one-third of cases of SLE. Psychiatric symptoms occur in 60% of cases: the excess is due to both psychological reactions to illness and corticosteroid side effects. The commonest presentations are acute organic states and neurotic disorders; schizophrenia-like syndromes are rare. Mental symptoms are seldom the first signs of SLE (which are usually fever, malaise and arthralgia). When present, psychiatric symptoms often fluctuate, usually remit within six weeks but may recur. The presence of cerebral vasculitis substantially worsens prognosis.

55. A

Dependent alcoholics suffer withdrawal symptoms as their blood alcohol level falls. The commonest feature is acute tremulousness in the morning, often with agitation, nausea, retching and sweating. These and more severe features such as fleeting hallucinations, fits and clouding of consciousness can be reduced by inpatient detoxification with chlormethiazole or benzodiazepine cover. Disulfiram (Antabuse) is used as an aid to willpower as it blocks oxidation of alcohol and produces unpleasant flushing, nausea and headache. Liver cirrhosis occurs in 10% of alcoholics. Intensive programmes of counselling are probably no more effective than brief advice.

56. B C

Retrograde amnesia is not a good prognostic factor. The duration of post-traumatic amnesia is more variable and is predictive of time to return to work, psychiatric disablement and personality change. Complete recall of the injury, particularly in an emotionally loaded setting, is predictive of neurotic disabilities. A personal or family history of mental disorder predicts later psychiatric incapacity. An increase in post-traumatic neurotic symptoms, intellectual and memory impairments and mortality is seen with increasing age. Compensation and litigation increase psychiatric sequelae, such symptoms being rare after injuries at sport or in the home where compensation is not payable. However settlement of compensation rarely leads to a significant resolution of psychiatric symptoms.

57. Post-Traumatic Stress Disorder (PTSD) following a disaster

- ☐ A affects primarily those with premorbid 'brittle' personalities
- ☐ B must by definition commence within 6 months of the traumatic event
- ☐ C is associated with alcohol and drug dependence
- ☐ D may provoke true hallucinations in clear consciousness
- ☐ E is characterised by regression to a child-like state

58. Lithium carbonate

- ☐ A should be discontinued in patients who develop hypothyroidism
- ☐ B commonly causes a 'pill rolling' tremor
- ☐ C toxicity often occurs when given concurrently with frusemide
- ☐ D serum levels should be monitored every three months
- ☐ E is teratogenic in the first trimester of pregnancy

59. The following are true about somatization disorder:

- ☐ A onset occurs usually after 30 years of age
- ☐ B the condition is more common in men than in women
- ☐ C the course tends to be fluctuating but chronic
- ☐ D anxiety and depression occur frequently
- ☐ E menstrual dysfunction in women is common

Answers overleaf

57. C D

Whilst a vulnerable personality increases risk of PTSD 50–80% of survivors of a disaster may develop the syndrome. Other risk factors include prior psychiatric disorder, extremes of age, concurrent physical disabilities and social depravation. PTSD usually develops sometime, possibly years, after the trauma and may mimic affective, anxiety or personality disorders. Features include reliving the trauma, dissociative flashbacks, illusions and hallucinations in full consciousness. Recurrent nightmares, intrusive recollections and avoidance of reminders of the trauma occur with intense distress if exposed to these and persistently increased autonomic arousal. Secondary problems include alcohol or drug dependence and marital discord. Psychodynamic theories invoke regression, repression, denial and undoing but child-like behaviour is not characteristic.

58. D E

5% of patients on long-term lithium develop hypothyroidism which is treated with thyroxine whilst lithium is continued. The 5 Hz 'pill rolling' tremor of Parkinsonism is a side effect of neuroleptic medication. Lithium induces a 7–16 Hz action tremor aggravated by anxiety and performance of fine motor movements. Thiazide diuretics increase lithium uptake in the proximal tubule, increase levels by 30–50% and potentially cause toxicity. Frusemide does not elevate serum lithium levels. Monitoring of lithium therapy involves three monthly serum lithium levels and six monthly thyroid and renal function tests. Lithium causes cardiac anomalies in the first trimester of pregnancy and particularly a 400-fold increase in Ebstein's anomaly of the tricuspid valve.

59. C D E

Somatization disorder is a chronic syndrome of multiple somatic symptoms that cannot be explained medically. It is associated with psychosocial distress and medical help-seeking. Diagnosis requires a history of several years duration. The onset occurs in early adulthood and rarely after 30 years of age. The belief that a person has been sickly most of their life is common. It is more common in women affecting 1–2% of all females. Interpersonal problems are prominent with anxiety and depression being the most prevalent psychiatric conditions. Menstrual symptoms, sexual indifference and frigidity, alcohol and drug abuse and antisocial personality disorder all occur more frequently. Whilst the disorder fluctuates, patients are rarely symptom free.

60. The following statements about mental retardation are true:

- ☐ A in mild retardation, subcultural influences are pre-eminent
- ☐ B there is an increased risk of psychosis
- ☐ C treatment for phenylketonuria should be continued for life
- ☐ D the features of cretinism are present at birth
- ☐ E neurofibromatosis is characteristically associated with self mutilation

61. In families of schizophrenic patients

- ☐ A there is an increased rate of depression
- ☐ B twins are more often mentally ill than non-twins
- ☐ C adoption does not reduce the genetic risk
- ☐ D alcoholism occurs more often than expected
- ☐ E when the proband develops the disease late in life, the risk to relatives is reduced

62. The following are essential elements of the alcohol dependence syndrome:

- ☐ A a compulsion to drink
- ☐ B an altered tolerance to alcohol
- ☐ C changing from beers to spirits
- ☐ D relief drinking
- ☐ E reinstatement after abstinence

Answers overleaf

60. A B

Most mental retardation is of uncertain aetiology. In mild retardation (IQ less than 50) there is a strong association with social handicap and low IQ in the family. Therefore, many cases represent the lower end of the intelligence spectrum ('subcultural' retardation). All psychiatric disorders are more common in mental retardation, although diagnosis is often difficult. Phenylketonuria requires dietary phenylalanine exclusion which can probably be ended after adolescence. Cretinism (congenital hypothyroidism) is not clinically detectable until six months. Lesch-Nyhan syndrome is an X-linked syndrome producing choreoathetoid movements and self mutilation. Neurofibromatosis is an autosomal dominant inherited disorder characterised by multiple tumours and vitiligo which only produces intellectual retardation in a minority of cases.

61. C D E

Family studies have shown that first degree relatives of schizophrenics have an increased rate of schizophrenia themselves (5–12% compared to 1% in the general population). Twin and adoption studies have confirmed the genetic contribution to aetiology. However twins per se have no greater risk than non-twins. Relatives also have higher rates of personality disorder and alcoholism but not depression or organic psychosis. Familial risk is less in late onset cases.

62. A B D E

Seven essential elements in the alcohol dependence syndrome have been described. These include a compulsion to drink (and continue drinking), primacy of drinking over other activities, an altered tolerance to alcohol, repeated withdrawal symptoms, drinking to relieve withdrawal (and particularly early morning drinking) and re-instatement after abstinence. The final element, a stereotyped pattern of drinking, refers to an unvarying daily pattern of drinking at regular intervals in order to ward off withdrawal symptoms. Whilst alcoholics often progress to stronger and cheaper sources of alcohol this is not an essential element of the syndrome.

63. Morbid jealousy (delusions of infidelity)

- ☐ A is associated with hypersexuality
- ☐ B is a significant cause of wife murder
- ☐ C is a recognised symptom of alcoholism
- ☐ D has a good prognosis when treated early
- ☐ E was attributed to unconscious homosexual urges by Freud

64. Recognised treatments for acute mania include

- ☐ A chlorpromazine
- ☐ B lithium carbonate
- ☐ C ECT – electroconvulsive therapy
- ☐ D carbamazepine
- ☐ E procyclidine

65. Features of delirium tremens (DTs) include

- ☐ A symptoms peaking 3–4 days after abstinence from alcohol
- ☐ B a mortality of 50%
- ☐ C Lilliputian hallucinations
- ☐ D hypomagnesaemia
- ☐ E insomnia

Answers overleaf

63. B C E

Pathological jealousy occurs in a wide range of psychiatric conditions notably personality disorder, paranoid psychosis and schizophrenia, depression and alcoholism. It is commoner in men, and is associated with erectile impotence. Freud believed it was caused by repression and reaction formation of homosexual drives. Morbid jealousy can be highly dangerous and is the cause of 10–20% of homicides in special hospitals (both male and female). Treatment of the primary disorder can be helpful but in most cases the symptom persists and marital separation may be the only solution.

64. A B C D

Acute mania is treated with a neuroleptic such as chlorpromazine. Immediate sedation is superseded by an antimanic effect over some weeks. Additional short-term sedation with a benzodiazepine is some-times required. Lithium is an antimanic agent with a similar latency of action and less efficacy than neuroleptics. It is sometimes used to augment the neuroleptic effect but occasional neurotoxicity has been reported. Carbamazepine has a mild antimanic effect but is used pri-marily as a prophylactic agent in patients intolerant to lithium or who have rapid cycling disorders (more than three episodes per year). ECT still has a role in drug resistant manic patients. Procyclidine is used to treat the Parkinsonian side-effects of neuroleptics.

65. A C D E

DTs are the most serious of the alcohol withdrawal phenomenon with a mortality of up to 5%. Prodromal symptoms occur shortly after abstinence but the full blown syndrome, characterised by vivid hallucinations, occurs 3–4 days later. Illusions and hallucinations are primarily visual but auditory and haptic hallucinations also occur. Lilliputian hallucinations may be accompanied by amusement and jocularity but an affect of apprehension and fear is more typical. Other symptoms include delusions, confusion, inattention, agitation, rest-lessness, tremor, autonomic overactivity and sleeplessness. Bio-chemical abnormalities include hypomagnesaemia, hypokalaemia and hypoglycaemia. Treatment is primarily with sedation, using chlordiazepoxide or chlormethiazole, adequate hydration, vitamin supplementation and anticonvulsant cover where there is a history of seizure.

66. The following drugs of abuse not infrequently induce paranoid psychoses:

☐ A lysergic acid diethylamide (LSD)

☐ B temazepam

☐ C heroin

☐ D volatile solvents

☐ E amphetamine

67. Tardive dyskinesia

☐ A is associated with previous brain damage

☐ B occurs in most patients on long-term neuroleptic treatment

☐ C is commoner in men

☐ D is associated with reduced life expectancy in severe schizophrenia

☐ E invariably improves on stopping the offending neuroleptic

68. The following Schneiderian 'first rank' symptoms are suggestive of a diagnosis of schizophrenia:

☐ A voices repeating the subjects thought out loud

☐ B thought broadcasting

☐ C Knight's move thinking

☐ D emotional blunting

☐ E emotional passivity

66. A D E

Hallucinogens including cannabis, mescaline, ecstasy, phencyclidine, psilocybin (magic mushrooms) and volatile solvents may induce a paranoid psychosis characterised by paranoid delusions and hallucinations without significant impairment of consciousness. CNS stimulants including amphetamines and cocaine and CNS depressants including alcohol, barbiturates and some high potency benzodiazepines have also been implicated. Temazepam withdrawal will rarely cause hallucinations but not a full blown paranoid psychosis. Heroin does not induce psychotic symptoms either in chronic use or during withdrawal.

67. D

Tardive dyskinesia is characterised by chewing, sucking and grimacing of the face and choreoathetoid movements. It occurs in about one fifth of patients receiving long-term treatment with neuroleptic medication such as phenothiazines or butyrophenones. Increased incidence is seen with females and increasing age but not brain damage or previous treatment with ECT. Few treatments are helpful and stopping the offending drug may produce paradoxical worsening. There is decreased life expectancy when functional psychosis and severe dyskinesia are both present.

68. A B E

Schneider considered symptoms of 'first rank' to be pathognomonic of schizophrenia in the absence of brain disease. They include specific auditory hallucinations (voices repeating or anticipating thoughts out loud, referring to the subject in the third person or maintaining a running commentary on the subjects thoughts or behaviour), thought interference (thought insertion, withdrawal and broadcasting), delusional perception (a form of primary delusion) and passivity phenomenon (the subject's feelings, impulses, acts and sensations appear under alien control). Schneider's 'second rank' symptoms included perplexity, emotional blunting and other kinds of hallucination and delusion. Bleuler, who coined the term 'schizophrenia' felt that loosening of associations, characterised by knights move thinking, was central to this disorder.

69. On general medical wards

☐ A at least one in ten patients has depression

☐ B medical students are better than nurses at detecting psychiatric disorder

☐ C about one in five patients have alcohol problems

☐ D medical outcome is affected by the presence of psychiatric disorder

☐ E most patients who have taken a drug overdose require inpatient assessment in a psychiatric unit

70. The following statements are true:

☐ A psychiatric abnormalities occur more commonly in multiple sclerosis than muscular dystrophy

☐ B in multiple sclerosis, euphoria is more frequent when disease-induced intellectual deficits are present

☐ C the intensity of depression in Parkinson's disease correlates with the severity of movement disorder

☐ D when depression occurs after a stroke, a lesion in the right parietal region should be strongly suspected

☐ E the most common psychiatric presentation of neurosyphilis is dementia

71. Monoamine oxidase inhibiting drugs (MAOIs) interact with

☐ A Bovril

☐ B tricyclic antidepressants

☐ C pethidine

☐ D phenelzine

☐ E phentolamine

Answers overleaf

69. A B C D

Hospital surveys have emphasised the frequency of psychiatric illness on general medical wards. The most common reason for admission is a drug overdose. Among patients admitted for other reasons, depression (10–25%) and alcohol abuse (15–30%) are very common. The diagnosis is often missed, especially if tearfulness or behaviour disturbances are not evident. This is important as continued psychiatric symptoms delay medical recovery. Research has shown that medical students can detect psychiatric cases more readily than house officers or ward nurses. About 10% of deliberate self-harm patients need inpatient psychiatric treatment.

70. A B C E

About 75% of patients with multiple sclerosis suffer from a psychiatric disorder at some stage. Euphoria and denial of disability are common associations of plaque-induced cognitive deficits, while depression is more often an early reaction to illness. Dementia and depression are also common in Parkinson's disease. There is a significant correlation between severity of depression and of the signs of Parkinson's disease. Strokes in the left frontal region are associated with depression; right parietal lesions often lead to denial of disability. Dementia and depression are both more common in neurosyphilis than the better known grandiose presentation (about 10% of cases).

71. A B C

Phenelzine is the most commonly prescribed monoamine oxidase inhibitor. Severe hypertensive crises may occur with tyramine-containing foods including cheese, meat and yeast extracts (like Bovril) and pickled herrings. Dangerous interactions may also occur with a wide range of drugs including ephedrine and phenyl-propanol-amine (proprietary cold remedies), methyldopa, opiates, barbiturates and tricyclic antidepressants. Some psychiatrists use combinations of MAOIs and tricyclic antidepressants to treat intractable depression, but this practice is dangerous in non-specialist hands. Phentolamine blocks alpha-adrenoceptors and is used to treat hypertensive crises induced by MAOI drugs.

72. Electroconvulsive treatment

- ☐ A is known to produce long-term memory impairment in patients when compared with untreated depressives
- ☐ B is not safe in patients over 80 years of age
- ☐ C is of no use in neurotic depression
- ☐ D is more successful in depression when delusions are present
- ☐ E has been validated in double blind trials

73. Predictors of poor outcome in schizophrenia include

- ☐ A early onset
- ☐ B asocial premorbid personality
- ☐ C family history of affective disorder
- ☐ D clear consciousness
- ☐ E negative symptoms

74. Puerperal psychosis

- ☐ A has been called 'maternity blues'
- ☐ B recurs in the majority of later pregnancies
- ☐ C is significantly increased after obstetric complications
- ☐ D should be managed by separation of mother and baby in most cases
- ☐ E may be accompanied by clouding of consciousness

Answers overleaf

72. D E

Recent double blind trials have confirmed the particular value of electroconvulsive therapy in depression especially when endogenous features or delusions are present. Although less used in other conditions, it is of value in neurotic depression, mania and schizophrenia. It causes brief memory disturbances after each application, especially when bilateral rather than unilateral electrodes are used. However, there is little evidence that permanent memory deficits occur. Age is no contraindication to treatment.

73. A B D E

Factors predictive of a poor outcome and chronic course in schizophrenia include an early age of onset, low socio-economic status, irregular occupational record, social adversity, a family history of schizophrenia, schizoid or asocial premorbid personality traits, low intelligence, lack of a lasting heterosexual relationship, absence of precipitating factors, insidious onset, longer duration of untreated psychosis, lack of clouding of consciousness or confusion, absence of a family history of affective disorder or an affective component to the illness, presence of primary negative symptoms, neurological signs and symptoms and a history of perinatal trauma.

74. E

Serious and minor mental disorders are considerably more common in the postpartum period. 'Maternity blues' is a self-limiting episode of mood lability occurring in about half of new mothers. Puerperal psychosis is far less common. No specific causative factors are known. A variety of presentations are possible, including acute organic reactions with clouding of consciousness. The development of supervised mother-and-baby units within psychiatric hospitals has avoided the need for separation and the consequent disruption of emotional 'bonding'. Psychosis recurs in about 20% of later pregnancies.

75. The following statements about benzodiazepines are true:

☐ A lorazepam has a longer duration of action than diazepam following a single dose

☐ B paradoxical disinhibition contraindicates continued use of benzodiazepines

☐ C nitrazepam is safe as a regularly prescribed hypnotic in the elderly

☐ D dependence is most likely with drugs that have a short elimination half-life

☐ E withdrawal symptoms are best treated with a sedative neuroleptic such as thioridazine

76. Delusions

☐ A only occur in schizophrenia

☐ B are not modified by contrary experience

☐ C are obsessions

☐ D are perceived as emanating from the external world

☐ E are false ideas

77. Delusions of persecution can occur in

☐ A paraphrenia

☐ B paranoid personality disorder

☐ C reactive depression

☐ D myxoedema

☐ E amphetamine abuse

Answers overleaf

75. A D

Lorazepam, a 'short-acting' benzodiazepine, has a longer distribution half-life (HLD) and thus a longer sedative effect following a single dose, but no active metabolites and a shorter elimination half-life (HLE; 10–20 hours) compared with the 'long-acting' benzodiazepine diazepam (HLE 30–100 hours). The HLE of nitrazepam, usually 18–36 hours, is longer in the elderly leading to drug accumulation, confusion, ataxia, falls and increased mortality. Paradoxical disinhibition may be treated with a dose reduction or increase. Dependence is increased by high doses, dose escalation, prolonged treatment, high potency drugs, drugs with a short HLE, and in patients with dependent personality traits. Withdrawal symptoms are best treated with a gradual reducing regime using a long-acting benzodiazepine.

76. B E

Delusions are morbid false beliefs, which occur in a wide range of psychoses including schizophrenia. Classically they are firmly held out of keeping with the patient's subculture and cannot be altered by reason or demonstration of their falsity. They often occur secondary to hallucinations, which are false percepts apparently in the external world. Obsessions are recurrent thoughts, images or impulses resisted by the patient who finds them both senseless and distressing, but recognises them as his own mental products.

77. A D E

Persecutory delusions are the leading feature of paraphrenia, a psychosis typically of elderly deaf, socially isolated women with premorbid schizoid or paranoid traits. Myxoedema can produce a variety of serious mental disorders, including paranoid psychosis. Amphetamine abuse frequently produces a psychotic disorder with paranoid delusions and hallucinations, which may remit rapidly with abstinence. Patients with paranoid personalities have a pervasive sense of being slighted or tricked which does not reach delusional intensity. Persecutory delusions occur in endogenous (psychotic) depression rather than reactive depression.

78. Characteristic features of endogenous depression include

    ☐ A incongruity of mood and thinking

    ☐ B early morning waking

    ☐ C failure to respond to chlorpromazine therapy

    ☐ D feelings of worthlessness

    ☐ E loss of libido

79. Factors which increase the risk of suicide include

    ☐ A advancing age

    ☐ B social class I

    ☐ C the presence of hopelessness

    ☐ D antisocial personality disorder

    ☐ E talking about suicidal ideas

80. Recognised features of depression in the elderly include

    ☐ A delusions of poverty

    ☐ B pseudodementia

    ☐ C a strong association with bereavement

    ☐ D agitated movements

    ☐ E retarded movements

Answers overleaf

78. B D E

In endogenous depression, there is persistent depression of mood, unreactive to circumstances. Characteristic symptoms include early morning waking, morning worsening of mood, feelings of guilt or worthlessness with decline in concentration, energy, appetite, interest and libido. Although tricyclic antidepressants and electroconvulsive therapy (ECT) are the treatments of choice, some cases, especially when agitation and/or delusions are present, respond to chlorpromazine alone. Affective incongruity is a feature of schizophrenia.

79. A B C D E

Suicide is commonest amongst elderly men, although rates amongst young men have been rising dramatically in recent years. Rates increase progressively through the married, never married, widowers and widows and the divorced. Suicide is increased amongst social classes I and V, individuals with a past history of suicide attempts, history of depression, alcohol abuse, drug abuse, schizophrenia or antisocial or borderline personality disorders. Feelings of hopelessness are an important predictor of immediate and long-term suicide risk. In most cases a warning is given before committing suicide with 2/3 expressing suicidal ideas to relatives and 1/3 expressing clear suicidal intent. 40% of suicide completers had consulted their GP in the previous week.

80. A B D E

Agitation and retardation both occur in a significant number of elderly depressives. When delusions are present, they usually have a depressive flavour (e.g. poverty or physical illness). A certain proportion have apparent cognitive deficits, which improve in parallel with the symptoms of depression: this is the commonest variety of 'pseudo-dementia'. Severe life events can precipitate depression in the elderly, but bereavement is less important as a cause of mental illness than in younger age groups.

81. Recognised features of anorexia nervosa include

☐ A increased plasma cortisol

☐ B frequent structural abnormalities of the hypothalamus

☐ C male hypersexuality

☐ D hypokalaemia

☐ E total loss of body hair

82. The following features suggest a normal bereavement reaction rather than depressive illness:

☐ A complaints of physical symptoms

☐ B emotional numbness

☐ C suicidal thoughts

☐ D searching behaviour

☐ E feelings of worthlessness

83. Confirmed risk factors for Alzheimer's disease include

☐ A head injury

☐ B smoking

☐ C aluminium

☐ D nose picking

☐ E Down's syndrome

Answers overleaf

81. A D

Anorexia nervosa is defined by self-induced weight loss, abnormal attitudes to food and body weight and amenorrhoea in women or loss of libido in men. There are many endocrine changes e.g. raised cortisol and growth hormone, and decreased gonadotrophins. However there is little evidence that it is a primary endocrinological disorder. Structural lesions are rarely discovered. Clinical features include lanugo, a type of downy hair found on the extremities. Induced vomiting and purging to reduce weight often result in hypokalaemia.

82. A B D

Bereavement reactions are normal, but share features in common with depression such as misery, tearfulness, insomnia, poor concentration and anorexia. Other features of depression such as psychomotor retardation, delusions, suicidal thinking and generalised loss of self-esteem only rarely occur in bereavement. Physical symptoms are more commonly reported by the bereaved. Most typically, three stages of grieving can be distinguished: an initial phase of emotional numbness and unreality; secondly a mourning phase of variable length which may include experiences of the presence or voice of the deceased and searching behaviour; finally there is gradual acceptance and resolution.

83. A D E

With the exception of the very elderly risk of Alzheimer's disease (AD) increases with age. Other well confirmed risk-factors include family history of Alzheimer's disease (particularly with early onset AD) and Down's syndrome. Recent findings have also implicated past inanition (later onset and sporadic AD), nervous breakdown (early onset AD), head injury (sporadic AD) and curiously nose picking (later onset AD). Alcohol is related to a small increase and smoking a small decrease in risk. At present evidence for aluminium in the aetiology and pathology of AD is considered circumstantial.

84. Panic attacks

- ☐ A usually have clearly identifiable precipitants
- ☐ B are important in the aetiology of social phobia
- ☐ C are characterised by an impending feeling of doom
- ☐ D are associated with mitral valve prolapse
- ☐ E respond primarily to behavioural interventions

85. Clinical features of delirium often include

- ☐ A decreased motor activity
- ☐ B diurnal variation in symptoms
- ☐ C perseveration
- ☐ D a catastrophic reaction
- ☐ E hallucinations

86. Recognized treatments for schizophrenia include

- ☐ A psychodynamic psychotherapy
- ☐ B clozapine
- ☐ C family therapy
- ☐ D Depo-Provera
- ☐ E psychosurgery

Answers overleaf

84. C D

Panic attacks are characterised by a sudden onset of extreme fear, an impending feeling of doom and somatic symptoms including tachycardia, palpitations, dyspnoea and sweating. Usually no precipitant is evident and attacks last 20–30 minutes. As many as 50% of patients have prolapse of one of the mitral valve leaflets, resulting in a midsystolic click on cardiac auscultation. The mainstay of treatment is antidepressants. Behavioural treatments may help with residual anxiety symptoms although controlled breathing and breathing into a bag are sometimes useful for attacks. Social phobia is a persistent fear of social appraisal and is not directly linked to panic disorder although most cases of agoraphobia are thought to be secondary to it.

85. A B C E

Delirium is an acute onset syndrome characterised by inattention and an impaired level of consciousness. Thinking is often disorganised and perseverative. Perceptual disturbances include misinterpretations, illusions and hallucinations. There is disturbance of the sleep-wake cycle with insomnia and daytime sleepiness. Psychomotor-activity may be increased or decreased. Disorientation and memory impairment are common. The patient has no insight during episodes of confusion and amnesia for the episode once it has resolved. A catastrophic reaction has been described in dementing patients which is characterised by marked agitation secondary to the subjective awareness of intellectual deficits under stressful circumstances.

86. B C

Treatment of schizophrenia is with long-term neuroleptic medication, often in depot form to ensure compliance. 70% respond to conventional neuroleptics and of the remainder 50% respond to the atypical anti-psychotic clozapine. Patients taking clozapine require regular blood monitoring in view of the risk of neutropenia and potentially fatal agranulocytosis. Family therapy may reduce relapse if relatives show high levels of 'expressed emotion'. Cognitive behavioural therapy may help patients with chronic symptoms and possibly also in the acute stages of the illness. Psychodynamic therapy is not useful and may precipitate a relapse in some patients. Psychosurgery is rarely used in intractable cases of depression and obsessive-compulsive disorder but has no role in the treatment of schizophrenia.

87. The following are true of affective disorders:

- ☐ A the male:female ratio in unipolar depression is 1:1
- ☐ B 70% of those with major depression receive treatment
- ☐ C bipolar disorder is more frequent amongst social class V
- ☐ D the prevalence of depression is reduced in non-Judeo-Christian cultures
- ☐ E lifetime prevalence of bipolar disorder is approximately 1%

88. Section 5(2) of the Mental Health Act (MHA) 1983

- ☐ A on medical wards should only be recommended by the duty psychiatrist
- ☐ B lasts for 72 hours
- ☐ C allows the appropriate psychiatric treatment to be commenced
- ☐ D allows surgical or medical treatments in the absence of patient consent
- ☐ E may be appealed against by the next of kin

89. The following drugs, pharmacological actions and clinical effects are related:

- ☐ A amitriptyline, alpha1-adrenergic receptor antagonism, postural hypotension
- ☐ B haloperidol, dopamine D1-receptor antagonism, antipsychotic effect
- ☐ C tranylcypromine, irreversible blockade of monoamine oxidase, 'the cheese reaction'
- ☐ D diazepam, GABA A agonism, anxiolytic effect
- ☐ E lithium, inhibitor of adenylyl cyclase activation by ADH, polyuria

Answers overleaf

87. E

Whilst depressive symptoms are very common lifetime prevalence of unipolar depression is about 6% and bipolar disorder 1%. The male: female ratio of unipolar depression is 1:2 whilst the sex ratio for bipolar disorder is approximately equal. Only 1 in 5 patients with major depression receive treatment, 1 in 50 enter hospital and 1 in 200 commit suicide. There are no consistent social class differences in the prevalence of unipolar depression although bipolar disorder may be slightly increased in social class I. There are no racial or cultural differences in the prevalence of depression although somatic symptoms are often prominent in third world settings and guilt in Judeo-Christian cultures.

88. B

Section 5(2) is an emergency holding order allowing detention of a patient, suspected of having a mental illness and of being a risk to themselves or others, for up to 72 hours. Recommendation is by the Responsible Medical Officer of the patient, or their nominated deputy. Only a consultant psychiatrist may nominate a deputy. Section 5(2) gives no rights to treatment without consent. No part of the MHA allows for non-psychiatric treatments without consent except when such treatment is for a physical disorder which is directly causing a psychiatric disorder. Where necessary treatment must be given under common law or section 62 of the MHA. Section 2 allows commencement of treatment. Section 3 is a 6 month treatment order. Neither the patient nor the next of kin have right to appeal against section 5(2).

89. A D E

Postural hypotension is a serious side-effect of tricyclic antidepressants, particularly in the elderly. Typical antipsychotics such as haloperidol have an antipsychotic action which is proportional to their antagonism of the dopamine D2 receptor. Tranylcypromine is a reversible inhibitor of MAO with some amphetamine-like properties. Ingestion of vaso-active amines, such as tyramine in cheese, may lead to a hyperadrenergic crisis. 50–70% of patients on long-term lithium develop polyuria, with 10% having an output exceeding 3 litres per day, thus qualifying as having nephrogenic diabetes insipidus. Lithium also inhibits adenylyl cyclase activation by TSH which is thought to be a factor in the production of drug-induced hypothyroidism or goitre.

90. Neuroleptic malignant syndrome

☐ A is characterised by hyperthermia and muscular rigidity

☐ B can occur when tricyclics alone are administered

☐ C most commonly occurs after haloperidol treatment

☐ D is usually fatal

☐ E responds to treatment with tetrabenzine

91. Significant side effects of selective serotonin reuptake inhibitors (SSRIs) include

☐ A anorgasmia

☐ B insomnia

☐ C sweating

☐ D dystonia

☐ E retention of urine

92. The following factors are significantly associated with episodes of deliberate self harm:

☐ A male unemployment

☐ B recent alcohol consumption

☐ C male sex

☐ D age over 40 years

☐ E epilepsy

Answers overleaf

90. A B C

Neuroleptic malignant syndrome is an uncommon but increasingly recognised side effect of neuroleptic administration. The syndrome is characterised by hyperthermia, muscle rigidity, a fluctuant conscious level, features of sympathetic discharge and, less consistently, dystonias and dyskinesias. It occurs at therapeutic doses. The most frequently implicated drug is haloperidol. Tricyclic antidepressant therapy and L-dopa withdrawal are occasional causes. There is no specific treatment. A significant minority of cases are fatal; the rest recover after drug withdrawal within one to three weeks.

91. A B C D

SSRIs are effective antidepressants with less sedative effect than tricyclics, few antimuscarinic effects and low cardiotoxicity. The most frequent side-effects are gastrointestinal (diarrhoea, nausea and vomiting) which are dose related. Restlessness, anxiety, insomnia and sweating may be marked initially. Side-effects also include anorexia, weight loss and allergic reactions including anaphylaxis (all more common with fluoxetine), convulsions (particularly with fluvoxamine), extrapyramidal reactions and a withdrawal syndrome (particularly with paroxetine), abnormalities of hepatic enzymes (particularly with fluvoxamine and sertraline) and sexual dysfunction including anorgasmia and ejaculatory failure in males (particularly with paroxetine and fluoxetine).

92. A B E

The most typical pattern of deliberate self harm is an impulsive drug overdose taken with mixed motives in a state of mental turmoil often by a young single girl after a quarrel or rejection. Important associations include recent life events, marital conflict, unemployment (in men), recent alcohol consumption (especially in men), personality disorder and epilepsy. In the year following an overdose, risk of suicide is 1–2% (100 times that of the general population).

93. Recognised features of Korsakov's syndrome include

☐ A denial of amnesia

☐ B impaired registration rather than retention

☐ C obsession with time

☐ D dysphasia

☐ E echopraxia

94. Structural imaging of the brain in schizophrenia has revealed

☐ A that degree of ventricular enlargement correlates with deficit symptoms

☐ B ventricular enlargement at onset

☐ C reduced volume of medial temporal lobe structures

☐ D widespread grey matter volume reductions

☐ E ventricular enlargement in the majority of patients when compared with unaffected siblings

95. The EEG in Creutzfeldt-Jacob disease (CJD)

☐ A allows a confident diagnosis to be made in the early stages

☐ B may show spike and wave discharges concurrent with myoclonic jerks

☐ C characteristically shows synchronous triphasic sharp wave complexes and suppression of cortical background activity

☐ D characteristically shows generalized low voltage fast activity or random slow activity progressing to a flat record

☐ E demonstrates characteristic changes which are commonly also evident in asymptomatic first degree relatives

Answers overleaf

93. A

Korsakov's syndrome is characterised by relatively circumscribed memory deficit where new information is registered but quickly forgotten. This results in disorientation in time. Patients usually have little awareness of their problem and make up stories (confabulate) to cover gaps in their memory. Associations include irritability, peripheral neuropathy and the Wernicke syndrome (ataxia, ophthalmoplegia and impaired consciousness). Common aetiologies are thiamine deficiency (due to alcohol abuse or gastrointestinal disease) and lesions of the mammillary bodies and medial thalamus. Echopraxia (automatic imitation of another's movements) is a symptom of catatonia.

94. B C D E

Studies report a significant increase in average lateral ventricle size in schizophrenics compared with normal controls, although with a marked overlap between the two populations. Third ventricle and cortical sulcal enlargement has also been reported. Medial temporal lobe structures appear reduced in volume, particularly on the left, and MRI has revealed widespread grey (but not white) matter volume deficits. Studies utilizing unaffected siblings as controls have demonstrated ventricular enlargement in the majority of patients. It has been demonstrated at illness onset and tends not to be progressive. There has been no consistent correlation shown between the degree of enlargement and symptoms although a relationship may exist with generalized cognitive deficits.

95. B C

The EEG in CJD initially shows diffuse or focal slowing which is nonspecific to this disorder. Later repetitive sharp waves or slow spike and wave discharges appear, which are bilaterally synchronous and may accompany myoclonic jerks. In the later stages of the disorder a characteristic pattern emerges of synchronous triphasic sharp wave complexes, superimposed on progressive suppression of cortical background activity. The sharp wave complexes become increasingly periodic at rates of one to two per second. These latter changes strongly suggest a diagnosis of CJD. Whilst EEG abnormalities found in epileptic patients are to some degree heritable those in CJD are not.

96. The following features are more likely to occur in depressive pseudodementia than in dementia:

☐ A recent onset of symptoms

☐ B extensive complaining by the patient about memory loss

☐ C worsening of cognitive symptoms in the evening

☐ D 'don't know' answers

☐ E past history of depression

97. Insight is usually present in the following forms of abnormal illness behaviour:

☐ A factitious disorder

☐ B Münchausen's syndrome

☐ C somatization disorder

☐ D conversion disorder

☐ E malingering

98. Twin studies have demonstrated the heritability of

☐ A schizophrenia

☐ B male homosexuality

☐ C juvenile delinquency

☐ D life events

☐ E unipolar depression

Answers overleaf

96. A B D E

The differential diagnosis of dementia and depression can be troublesome when cognitive symptoms complicate the latter. In depression, careful questioning will typically elicit more recent onset and more rapid progression of symptoms and possibly a past history or family history of depression. Features of the mental state suggesting depression include complaints about memory loss, 'don't know' rather than 'near miss' answers to specific questions and concurrent depressive symptoms. All these features are less common in dementia. In depression there is morning worsening of mood while in dementia there is evening worsening of confusion.

97. A B E

Factitious disorder is characterised by an intentional production of physical or psychological symptoms with an evident psychological need to assume the sick role. The disorder is best known as Münchausen's syndrome and patients are very difficult to manage, often discharging themselves when confronted with their factitious behaviour. In malingering there is an obvious, recognizable environmental goal in producing symptoms, beyond assuming the sick role. Somatization disorder is characterised by multiple physical complaints. Despite the absence of any physical disorder which would explain them the patient genuinely believes himself to be ill. Hysterical conversion disorders are characterised by physical, often neurological, symptoms which produce evident primary and secondary gain, but which are not consciously simulated by the patient.

98. A B D E

Heritability of schizophrenia is between 63% and 80%, with no common environmental effect. It is also substantial in bipolar disorder, and to a lesser extent unipolar depression. With decreasing severity of illness the genetic effect in 'neurotic' disorders decreases, whilst a common environmental component becomes more important. Proneness to 'life events' also has a genetic component and implicated life events are those felt to have been influenced by 'hazard prone' individuals. Male homosexuality has a heritability of between 31% and 74%. Genetic factors significantly influence adult criminality, with pairwise concordance rates of 51% in monozygous twins and 22% in dizygous twins, contrasting with rates for juvenile delinquency (monozygous 87% and dizygous 72%), which suggest an insignificant genetic effect.

99. Huntington's chorea

- ☐ A is caused by an X-linked gene
- ☐ B is the commonest cause of choreiform movements first occurring in the second half of life
- ☐ C is associated with decreased glutamic acid decarboxylase (GAD)
- ☐ D particularly affects the cerebral cortex and basal ganglia
- ☐ E causes rapidly progressive dementia in the majority of cases

100. The following features are found in the majority of cases of Down's syndrome:

- ☐ A IQ between 20 and 50
- ☐ B death before the age of 50 years
- ☐ C congenital heart disease
- ☐ D behaviour disorder
- ☐ E flat occiput

Answers overleaf

99. C D

Huntington's chorea is an uncommon autosomal dominant disorder affecting 4–7 per 100,000 of the population. Senile and drug-induced choreas are much more frequently encountered. Anatomically, the frontal lobes and the caudate nucleus are most severely affected by neuronal loss and gliosis. Decreased concentrations of the inhibitory transmitter gamma-amino-butyric acid (GABA) and its enzyme glutamic acid decarboxylase (GAD) are usually detected. Dementia is usual although not invariable and progresses slowly over five to fifteen years.

100. A B E

Down's syndrome is the commonest known cause of moderate or severe subnormality (IQ less than 50). Characteristic features include small mouth with furrowed tongue and high palate, flat occiput, eyes with oblique palpebral fissures and epicanthic folds, hypotonia, short broad hands with curved little finger and a single palmar crease. Congenital heart disease (especially septal defects) occurs in one fifth of cases. Behaviour disorders are less common than in many syndromes of mental handicap. Despite improvements in care, death in early or middle life is still usual.

NEUROLOGY: REVISION CHECKLIST

Abnormalities of brain & cerebral circulation

- ☐ Dementia/Alzheimer's
- ☐ Lateral medullary/circulatory syndromes
- ☐ Head injury
- ☐ Benign intracranial hypertension/brain tumour
- ☐ Hemiplegic migraine
- ☐ Parietal lobe/frontal cortical lesions
- ☐ Temporal lobe epilepsy
- ☐ Central pontine myelinolysis
- ☐ Cerebral abscess
- ☐ EEG
- ☐ Encephalitis
- ☐ Intracranial calcification
- ☐ Normal pressure hydrocephalus
- ☐ Subdural haematoma
- ☐ Transient ischaemic attacks

Spinal cord and peripheral nerve anatomy & lesions

- ☐ Innervation of hand muscles
- ☐ Posterior nerve root/spinal ganglia lesions
- ☐ Dorsal interosseous nerve
- ☐ Guillain-Barré
- ☐ Median nerve
- ☐ Cervical spondylosis
- ☐ Paraesthesia
- ☐ Pyramidal tracts
- ☐ Radial nerve
- ☐ Sciatic nerve lesions
- ☐ Spinal cord lesions

Cranial nerve anatomy & lesions

- ☐ Cranial nerve lesions
- ☐ Facial nerve
- ☐ Third nerve palsy/pupillary reflex
- ☐ Bulbar palsy
- ☐ Internuclear ophthalmoplegia
- ☐ 4th nerve palsy

Dyskinesias

- ☐ Ataxia
- ☐ Benign essential tremor
- ☐ Dyskinesia
- ☐ Parkinson's disease

Muscular disorders

- ☐ Duchenne muscular dystrophy
- ☐ Myotonic dystrophy

Miscellaneous

- ☐ Multiple sclerosis
- ☐ Nystagmus
- ☐ Lumbar puncture/CSF
- ☐ Vertigo/dysarthria
- ☐ Autonomic neuropathy
- ☐ CNS involvement in AIDS
- ☐ Headache
- ☐ Pseudofits

PSYCHIATRY: REVISION CHECKLIST

Psychotic disorders

- ☐ Depression/insomnia
- ☐ Schizophrenia
- ☐ Mania
- ☐ Hallucinations/delusions

Anxiety states/compulsive disorders

- ☐ Neurosis/psychogenic/conversion
- ☐ Obsessional/compulsive disorders

Eating disorders

- ☐ Anorexia nervosa
- ☐ Bulimia

Other cognitive disorders

- ☐ Dementia
- ☐ Acute confusional states

Miscellaneous

- ☐ Alcohol dependency
- ☐ Narcolepsy

NEUROLOGY REVISION INDEX

Numbers refer to question numbers.

PSYCHIATRY REVISION INDEX

Numbers refer to question numbers.